Lean Diet:

6 Weeks to Become a Lean Green Eating Machine!

Table of Contents

Introduction

Making a major dietary change isn't easy and choosing this book or others like it is a great first step. Inside you will learn everything there is to know about the lean diet and how it can help you lose weight and build muscle mass at the same time.

This book contains proven steps and strategies designed to ensure you make the most out of your dieting experience in one of the healthiest, and least restrictive diets around. That doesn't mean it is for everyone, however, which is why it is important to always consult a dietitian or healthcare professional before making any major dietary changes. This is always recommended to ensure you aren't accidentally doing yourself more harm than good. With that in mind, get ready to start on the road to a healthier and happier you!

Thanks again for downloading this book, I hope you enjoy it!

Chapter 1: All About the Lean Diet

Unlike many diet plans that are all about skewing your diet towards one extreme or another or counting the caloric content of every single thing you eat, the Lean diet is all about moderation. A good lean meal is part protein, part healthy carbohydrates and part healthy fats; and more importantly, it is low in processed ingredients or excessive sugar. The only thing you need to worry about is how natural an individual piece of food is, the rest takes care of itself.

Foods that are encouraged on the lean diet are those that are broadly considered clean, that is, those that are not processed which means they are free of chemical colorings, flavorings or textures, preservatives and additives. As a general rule, the higher the percentage of processed ingredients something has, the less nutrition it actually has as well. Your goal should be to moderate your carbohydrate intake to reasonable levels and decrease your sugar intake drastically as well. Outside of the general food restrictions, the lean diet can be broken down into several main principles.

Account for what you eat
Aside from eating as many naturally occurring foods as possible, the other biggest thing to consider when striving to follow a lean lifestyle is that, while not actively counting calories, you do need to be aware of what is going into and being burned up by your body. This is determined by your metabolism which is a combination of how you digest food, which accounts for roughly 10 percent of your total metabolism. You can improve your general digestion rate by eating more protein as a greater portion of protein calories are burned while swallowing as opposed to other types of food.

It is likewise important to make a conscious effort to get up and move more, as the amount you move is directly related to roughly 30 percent of your total metabolism. This is one of the reasons it is so important to exercise regularly when following the lean diet as discussed in chapter 2. The rest of your metabolism is committed to automated bodily functions which is why simply cutting your caloric intake indiscriminately never really works. Instead, this simply leaves you with less energy overall which slows your metabolism and makes it more likely for your body to hang on to every calorie.

When it comes to eating regularly, your thoughts are also going to have to change. When following a lean lifestyle, you should plan on eating 3 regular sized meals as well as two protein rich snacks each and every day. This will help your metabolism stay at a more consistent rate by preventing both blood sugar and insulin levels from spiking and crashing as it common with the standard 3 meal cycle. When it comes to portion sizes, you should limit proteins to those the size of your open hand and carbohydrates to the size of a first. Eat as many healthy vegetables as you like.

Find better fuel
Following a lean lifestyle means that some 80 percent of the food you each should have no ingredient labels. This means things like beans, potatoes, vegetables, fruits, seeds, nuts, milk, eggs, fish and grass-fed animals. 10 percent should be devoted strictly to the additional protein that you will need in order to make the most of the lean diet (1 gram per pound of body weight) this generally means protein powders which are fine as long as they contain very little sugar. The remaining 10 percent should also be made up of foods that you don't eat regularly, to expand your nutrient portfolio as well as your horizons.

Know your targets
To follow the lean diet successfully, you will need to consume protein for approximately 30 percent of your total daily intake. Protein is beneficial for losing weight because it makes you feel full longer, while also improving your metabolism and maintaining your muscle

mass. Depending on the amount of weight you are interested in losing, you will want to aim for between .5 and .7 grams of fat per pound of body weight. The more you have to lose, the greater the amount of fat per pound you will want to start with.

These fats should all be of the healthy variety which includes things like palm oil, avocados, eggs, lard, chicken fat, coconut oil, clarified butter, ghee and beef tallow. Fats to avoid include canola oil, blended oils, saturated fats and most salad dressing. A higher percentage of healthy fat in your diet will mean a decrease in the overall number of carbohydrates you consume which means your body will burn fat for energy instead.

Do the math
With these numbers in mind, all you have to do is plug in your own specifics and figure out the details that are right for you. From there, all you need to do is figure out how many calories you are burning as you exercise and make a point of consuming a smaller amount each day than what you expend. Once you have a series of concrete goals in mind you will find that it is much easier to get started as there are clear metrics for success and failure in place.

The meal plan outlined in chapters 4 through 9 was designed with a 165 lbs. individual in mind who is following the exercise guide outlined in chapter 2. Make sure to alter it to fit your specifics with that in mind. Consider the recipes outlined within as a guidebook to indicate the sorts of meals you should be looking for when it comes to planning out the meal plan that works for you.

Chapter 2: Exercise and the Lean Diet

One of the best benefits of the lean diet is that, in addition to being extremely healthy, it naturally puts the body in a state that makes it easier to shed fat and build muscle. It is important to build on these natural proclivities by committing to an exercise program similar to the one outlined below.

The following exercise plan is for those who are already at a moderate to good level of fitness. If you aren't quite there yet, simply choose a few exercises from the list each day and add additional exercises as you feel you are able. Remember, it is important to choose weights that allow you to complete the number of sets and repetitions listed with only a moderate amount of struggle.

If the exercises are too easy, increase the weight being used, if they are too hard, go down a weight instead. It is important to always use the right weights for you, if you go too light on the weight then you are simply wasting time, commit to exercising regularly or you are cheating yourself out of the true efficacy of the lean diet. Don't forget to warm up for approximately 10 minutes before starting your training for the day and don't underestimate the benefits of a cool down period as well.

Week 1 Day 1 Biceps and Back
- *Bent over twin dumbbell row:* Do 2 sets of between 10 and 12 repetitions if you can, do at least 1 set if possible.

- *Pullups:* Do 2 sets of between 10 and 12 repetitions if you can, do at least 1 set if possible.

- *Standing Wide Grip Barbell Curl:* Do 2 sets of between 10 and 12 repetitions if you can, do at least 1 set if possible.

- *Alternating Dumbbell Bicep Curl:* Do 2 sets of between 10 and 12 repetitions if you can, do at least 1 set if possible.

- *Elliptical:* 1 or 2 minutes on an easy resistance, between 1 and 3 minutes on a moderate resistance, between 1 and 3 minutes on a difficult resistance, alternate between resistance level 2 and resistance level 3 for between 8 and 10 minutes, between 1 and 3 minutes on medium resistance and between 1 and 2 minutes on easy resistance. Shoot for between 25 and 30 minutes' total.

Tips

- It is important to always use the correct form to make sure you get the most effective, and safest workout possible.

- Ideally, you want each repetition to take about 2 seconds to complete the lift portion and no more than 3 seconds to return to the original position.

- Never swing the weights, always remain complete control. This means not letting gravity do the work on the return to the starting positon.

- Rest as long as you need to catch your breath, don't milk it, however, and work to maintain a steady heart rate.

Week 1 Day 2 Triceps, Shoulders, Chest

- *Medium Grip Barbell Bench Press:* Do 2 sets of between 10 and 12 repetitions if you can, do at least 1 set if possible.

- *Twisting Dumbbell Fly Inclines*: Do 2 sets of between 10 and 12 repetitions if you can, do at least 1 set if possible.

- *Sitting Dumbbell Press:* Do 2 sets of between 10 and 12 repetitions if you can, do at least 1 set if possible.

- *Lateral Side Raises:* Do 2 sets of between 10 and 12 repetitions if you can, do at least 1 set if possible.

- *Overhead Triceps Press:* Do 2 sets of between 10 and 12 repetitions if you can, do at least 1 set if possible.

- *Dips:* Do 2 sets of between 10 and 12 repetitions if you can, do at least 1 set if possible.

Tips

- When warming up, it is important to get your tendons and muscles heated up and elastic enough for the trials ahead. Always warm up and cool down to help prevent injury.

- When lifting your goal should be to simulate your muscles, not to annihilate them. Lifting an overly heavy weight will actually break down your muscles, not help them get stronger. Lift the right amount and you will see steadier progress over time.

- When it comes to resting, try and rest a minute or less between arms or abs sets and no more than 2 minutes between leg sets for the best results.

Week 1 Day 3 Cardio Only

- *Elliptical:* 1 or 2 minutes on an easy resistance, between 1 and 3 minutes on a moderate resistance, between 1 and 3 minutes on a difficult resistance, alternate between resistance level 2 and resistance level 3 for between 8 and 10 minutes, between 1 and 3 minutes on medium resistance and between 1 and 2 minutes on easy resistance. Shoot for between 25 and 30 minutes' total.

Week 1 Day 4 Abs and Legs

- *Barbell Squats:* Do 2 sets of between 10 and 12 repetitions if you can, do at least 1 set if possible.

- *Lunges with Dumbbells:* Do 2 sets of between 10 and 12 repetitions if you can, do at least 1 set if possible.

- *Reverse Leg Curls:* Do 2 sets of between 10 and 12 repetitions if you can, do at least 1 set if possible.

- *Stiff Leg Deadlift Barbell:* Do 2 sets of between 10 and 12 repetitions if you can, do at least 1 set if possible.

- *Sitting Calf Raise:* Do 2 sets of between 10 and 12 repetitions if you can, do at least 1 set if possible.

- *Calf Raises Standing:* Do 2 sets of between 10 and 12 repetitions if you can, do at least 1 set if possible.

- *Crunches:* Do 2 sets of between 10 and 12 repetitions if you can, do at least 1 set if possible.

You are likely going to be feeling a bit sore after hitting the legs so hard today so it is extremely important that you stretch after you have finished working out. Do yourself a favor and plan for a little extra sleep tonight as well.

Week 1 Day 5 Biceps and Back

- *Pullups:* Do 2 sets of between 10 and 12 repetitions if you can, do at least 1 set if possible.

- *Dumbbell Rows:* Do 2 sets of between 10 and 12 repetitions if you can, do at least 1 set if possible.

- *Back Extensions:* Do 2 sets of between 10 and 12 repetitions if you can, do at least 1 set if possible.

- *Concentration curls:* Do 2 sets of between 10 and 12 repetitions if you can, do at least 1 set if possible.

- *Preacher Curls:* Do 2 sets of between 10 and 12 repetitions if you can, do at least 1 set if possible.

- *Elliptical:* 1 or 2 minutes on an easy resistance, between 1 and 3 minutes on a moderate resistance, between 1 and 3 minutes on a difficult resistance, alternate between resistance level 2 and resistance level 3 for between 8 and 10 minutes, between 1 and 3 minutes on medium resistance and between 1 and 2 minutes on easy resistance. Shoot for between 25 and 30 minutes' total.

Week 1, Day 6 Cardio

- *Elliptical:* 1 or 2 minutes on an easy resistance, between 1 and 3 minutes on a moderate resistance, between 1 and 3 minutes on a difficult resistance, alternate between resistance level 2 and resistance level 3 for between 8 and 10 minutes, between 1 and 3 minutes on medium resistance and between 1 and 2 minutes on easy resistance. Shoot for between 25 and 30 minutes' total.

Week 1, Day 7 Triceps, Shoulders, Chest

- *Medium Grip Incline Barbell Bench Press:* Do 2 sets of between 10 and 12 repetitions if you can, do at least 1 set if possible.

- *Butterfly:* Do 2 sets of between 10 and 12 repetitions if you can, do at least 1 set if possible.

- *Lateral Side raise:* Do 2 sets of between 10 and 12 repetitions if you can, do at least 1 set if possible.

- *Sitting Dumbbell Press:* Do 2 sets of between 10 and 12 repetitions if you can, do at least 1 set if possible.

- *Pushdown for Triceps:* Do 2 sets of between 10 and 12 repetitions if you can, do at least 1 set if possible.

- *Overhead Barbell Triceps Extensions:* Do 2 sets of between 10 and 12 repetitions if you can, do at least 1 set if possible.

Week 2, Day 1 Abs and Legs

- *Leg Press:* Do 2 sets of between 10 and 12 repetitions if you can, do at least 1 set if possible.

- *Leg Extensions:* Do 2 sets of between 10 and 12 repetitions if you can, do at least 1 set if possible.

- *Sitting Leg Curl:* Do 2 sets of between 10 and 12 repetitions if you can, do at least 1 set if possible.

- *Dumbbell Deadlift:* Do 2 sets of between 10 and 12 repetitions if you can, do at least 1 set if possible.

- *Sitting Calf Raise:* Do 2 sets of between 10 and 12 repetitions if you can, do at least 1 set if possible.

- *Crunches:* Do 2 sets of between 10 and 12 repetitions if you can, do at least 1 set if possible.

- *Hanging Leg Raise:* Do 2 sets of between 10 and 12 repetitions if you can, do at least 1 set if possible.

Week 2, Day 2 Cardio
- *Elliptical:* 1 or 2 minutes on an easy resistance, between 1 and 3 minutes on a moderate resistance, between 1 and 3 minutes on a difficult resistance, alternate between resistance level 2 and resistance level 3 for between 8 and 10 minutes, between 1 and 3 minutes on medium resistance and between 1 and 2 minutes on easy resistance. Shoot for between 25 and 30 minutes' total.

Week 2, Day 3 Biceps and Back
- *Single Arm Dumbbell Rows:* Do 2 sets of between 10 and 12 repetitions if you can, do at least 1 set if possible.

- *Cable Pulldowns:* Do 2 sets of between 10 and 12 repetitions if you can, do at least 1 set if possible.

- *Barbell Deadlifts:* Do 2 sets of between 10 and 12 repetitions if you can, do at least 1 set if possible.

- *Alternating Bicep Curls:* Do 2 sets of between 10 and 12 repetitions if you can, do at least 1 set if possible.

- *Standing Cable Curls:* Do 2 sets of between 10 and 12 repetitions if you can, do at least 1 set if possible.

- *Elliptical:* 1 or 2 minutes on an easy resistance, between 1 and 3 minutes on a moderate resistance, between 1 and 3 minutes on a difficult resistance, alternate between resistance level 2 and resistance level 3 for between 8 and 10 minutes, between 1 and 3 minutes on medium resistance and between 1 and 2 minutes on easy resistance. Shoot for between 25 and 30 minutes' total.

Week 2, Day 4 Shoulders, Triceps and Chest
- *Medium Grip Barbell Bench Press:* Do 2 sets of between 10 and 12 repetitions if you can, do at least 1 set if possible.

- *Dumbbell Flies (Inclined):* Do 2 sets of between 10 and 12 repetitions if you can, do at least 1 set if possible.

- *Seated Rear Deltoid Muscle Raise:* Do 2 sets of between 10 and 12 repetitions if you can, do at least 1 set if possible.

- *Triceps Dips:* Do 2 sets of between 10 and 12 repetitions if you can, do at least 1 set if possible.

Week 2, Day 5 Cardio
- *Elliptical:* 1 or 2 minutes on an easy resistance, between 1 and 3 minutes on a moderate resistance, between 1 and 3 minutes on a difficult resistance, alternate between resistance level 2 and resistance level 3 for between 8 and 10 minutes, between 1 and 3 minutes on medium resistance and between 1 and 2 minutes on easy resistance. Shoot for between 25 and 30 minutes' total.

Week 2, Day 6 Abs and Legs
- *Barbell Squats:* Do 2 sets of between 10 and 12 repetitions if you can, do at least 1 set if possible.

- *Lunges with Dumbbells:* Do 2 sets of between 10 and 12 repetitions if you can, do at least 1 set if possible.

- *Sitting Leg Curls:* Do 2 sets of between 10 and 12 repetitions if you can, do at least 1 set if possible.

- *Barbell Deadlifts:* Do 2 sets of between 10 and 12 repetitions if you can, do at least 1 set if possible.

- *Sitting Calf Raises:* Do 2 sets of between 10 and 12 repetitions if you can, do at least 1 set if possible.

- *Calf Raises While Standing:* Do 2 sets of between 10 and 12 repetitions if you can, do at least 1 set if possible.

- *Crunches:* Do 2 sets of between 10 and 12 repetitions if you can, do at least 1 set if possible.

- *Leg Raises While Hanging:* Do 2 sets of between 10 and 12 repetitions if you can, do at least 1 set if possible.

Week 2, Day 7

- *Biceps and Back:* Do 2 sets of between 10 and 12 repetitions if you can, do at least 1 set if possible.

- *Pullups:* Do 2 sets of between 10 and 12 repetitions if you can, do at least 1 set if possible.

- *Back Extensions:* Do 2 sets of between 10 and 12 repetitions if you can, do at least 1 set if possible.

- *Concentrated Curls:* Do 2 sets of between 10 and 12 repetitions if you can, do at least 1 set if possible.

- *Barbell Curls:* Do 2 sets of between 10 and 12 repetitions if you can, do at least 1 set if possible.

- *Elliptical:* 1 or 2 minutes on an easy resistance, between 1 and 3 minutes on a moderate resistance, between 1 and 3 minutes on a difficult resistance, alternate between resistance level 2 and resistance level 3 for between 8 and 10 minutes, between 1 and 3 minutes on medium resistance and between 1 and 2 minutes on easy resistance. Shoot for between 25 and 30 minutes' total.

Keep it up

There you have it, the basic outline of the type of exercise plan you should get into the habit of following regularly. For the next two weeks, try and focus on improving the number of repetitions you complete each set and decreasing the extra time you spend resting. The third set of two weeks should then be focused on maximizing your repetitions even more, with the goal of looking to increase the number of sets you are doing by 1, starting at the 8-week mark.

Remember, if you are anxious to build muscle as quickly as possible, the best way to do so is to aim for at least 10 repetitions with each set. This is the magic number when it comes to activating as much of your muscle tissue as possible. From that point on, each repetition you do is actively training your muscles as effectively as possible. Keep pushing yourself to do 1 more repetitions and the number of repetitions you can do will slowly but surely skyrocket.

While the first few weeks of regular exercise will likely lead to plenty of real results right off the bat, especially when coupled with the diet discussed in the following chapters, it is important to understand that you will not reach your goals overnight. Depending on how much work you have to do, it could be months, or maybe even years before you get the body of your dreams. While this may seem like an unfair slog, it is important to remember how long it took you to reach the point you were at before you started following a lean lifestyle and cut yourself some slack.

It is important to have a realistic level of expectation when it comes to the results you will see on the lean diet and not discount the methodical, if relatively unimpressive weekly returns that eating lean will bring you. However, week after week and month after month, if you stick with it, not only will you feel healthier and more full of energy than you ever thought possible, but you will eventually look in the mirror and hardly recognize the person looking back. Getting healthy is a marathon, not a sprint, slow and steady wins the race every time.

Chapter 3: Tips for Success and Mistakes to Avoid

Substitutions

When you first begin transitioning to a lean lifestyle, you may find that you routinely get cravings for specific types of foods that are now off of the table. One of the biggest reasons that many people fail to start a new diet once they have committed to it is they don't account for just how addictive many types of processed foods really are. Don't fall victim to the lure of unhealthy options, have a plan in place by keeping the following list in mind. The next time you get a craving, consider countering it in the following ways.

- Replace chocolate ice cream with chocolate flavored fat free Greek yogurt.

- Replace an ice cream sundae with frozen yogurt topped with fruit.

- Replace cheese doodles with non-processed cubes of actual cheese for a snack full of healthy fats.

- Replace chips and dip with vegetables and hummus.

- Replace a candy bar with a healthy protein bar.

- Replace potato chips with a small amount of air popped popcorn.

- Replace a cheese burger with a soy or black bean patty.

- Replace other salty favorites with healthy nut options instead.

In general, it is important to stay away from anything that is high in trans fats, sodium, sugar and hydrogenated oil. It is also important to try and limit your alcohol and soda and instead focus on drinking at least 12 cups of water per day. Both coffee and tea are acceptable as long as they are consumed black and not to excess.

Transitioning to a lean lifestyle

Unlike transitioning to many other diets, transitioning to a lean lifestyle can be relatively painless, depending on how committed you already are to eating primarily natural foods. If, however, you are heavily committed to processed foods, then you are in for an unfortunate couple of weeks. The high levels of fat and sugar that are found in most processed foods these days make many of them literally addictive.

This means that when you commit to cleaning out your refrigerator and going cold turkey with healthy alternatives you will feel the physical symptoms of withdrawal, the same as those detoxing from harmful drugs or alcohol. As such, you can either prepare for an unpleasant week or so whereby your body can experience flu like symptoms, or you can go cool turkey and try and wean yourself off of the unhealthier parts of your diet slowly to make the transition less painful.

If you make the decision to wean yourself off slowly, it is important to not try and follow the lean diet partially, and instead to work until you have gotten your sugar and fat consumption to a healthier point before committing to the new diet completely. Starting the lean diet partially is not recommended because of the dedication required when it comes to certain protein and healthy fat levels, something that cannot be guaranteed when processed foods are still in the mix. Don't give yourself an out when it comes to bailing on your new lifestyle prematurely, give it your all when you are in a position to do so.

Once you are ready to get started, it is important to do yourself a favor for later and take a number of "before" photographs and measurements to aid yourself in committing long term by proving yourself the opportunity to look back on how far you have come. This means you will want to weigh yourself on a scale as well as determine your current level of muscle mass and body fat. Don't forget to measure your shoulders, chest, waist, calves, thighs and arms for the best results.

While it may be difficult to look at yourself in such an analytical light, now, you will be happy in a few weeks' time when you have a baseline to compare your progress to. Write down your current measurements and put them someplace you will see them every morning, write down the new ones each time you take them and keep them in the same place. This visual representation of the timeline will make transitioning to the new lifestyle successfully much more manageable.

Sticking with a lean lifestyle
Once you have followed the outline provided in this book, you will need to make an effort set new goals for yourself if you hope to continue with the lean lifestyle in the long term. When choosing goals, it is important to choose those that are realistic to keep yourself from getting discouraged. This means losing between 1 and 1.5 lbs. per week in the long term while continuing to build muscle. Anything more than that is not just unrealistic, it is downright dangerous.

Instead of focusing on specific numbers on the scale, focus on increasing your number of repetitions or sets while exercising or how a specific item of clothing fits at different points in your journey. It is important to always have external factors working to push you in the right direction to keep your mind focused on the type of thought that will ensure you keep exercising regularly long enough for it to become a lifelong habit.

Likewise, it is important to be realistic about the fact that, now and then, you won't have the impregnable willpower required to stop yourself from eating something so delicious and so bad for you. If the healthy alternatives discussed above aren't enough to take your mind off of that one special something, it is instead a good idea to try and mitigate the damage as much as possible. Have 1, cupcake, not 20.

As long as you don't go crazy, there's no reason to feel guilty about the splurge afterwards, instead, take the time to think about how much healthier you are compared to when you started. The most important thing in these splurge scenarios is to not let the fact that you have gotten a little off book be the reason that you fall back into bad behavior. There is nothing wrong will a little splurge now and then, as long as you have the willpower to keep it an occasional thing.

Consider Carb Cycling
If you are looking to take the weight loss potential of your new lean lifestyle to the next level, you can consider adding carb cycling into the mix as well. Carb cycling is a separate type of dieting whereby you alternate the amount of carbohydrates you eat on certain days. Like the lean lifestyle, carb cycling focuses on eating clean foods and eating three large meals per day as well as two protein-rich snacks. It also promotes natural weight loss and lean muscle growth while improving your metabolism, all things that a lean lifestyle promotes as well.

Carb cycling works by ensuring you stock up on carbohydrates on your higher carbohydrate days to ensure you have the fuel you need to get you through the low carbohydrate days. Over time, this creates a scenario whereby your body starts burning a higher amount of calories on the higher carbohydrate days and then slowly begins to burn that higher amount of calories on the lower carbohydrate days which eventually become more and more frequent.

To get started carb cycling, you can start out alternating the days you can eat a higher amount of carbohydrates and the days you eat a smaller amount of carbohydrates and on each of the high amount of carbohydrates days you can eat a splurge item as long as you don't eat it in the evening. Starting on Monday, alternate between low and high carbohydrate days and allow both Saturday and Sunday to be higher carbohydrate days. On the low carbohydrate days, stick with 15 net grams of carbohydrates per day. Net carbohydrates are your total number of carbohydrates minus the amount of fiber you consume in the same day.

From there you can move on to a more standard, low/high split with Sunday being the only day that allows a splurge item. If you are looking to lose weight even faster you can double, or even triple up the ratio of lower carb to higher carb days as well.

When it comes to syncing carb cycling up with the rest of your schedule, it is important to ensure that the days you are eating the most carbohydrates are also the days that you are exercising the most stringently. Your body naturally needs more carbohydrates when exercising heavily anyway, might as well start putting all those extra carbs to good use right away. Don't forget to decrease the amount of healthy fat you eat on high carbohydrate days to balance things out.

Remember, just because you have the carbohydrate green light, doesn't mean you can eat unhealthy carbohydrates, instead you should stick to those that are complex which generate energy over a longer period of time. Reach for sweet potatoes, brown rice and dark, leafy vegetables and whatever you do, avoid high fructose corn syrup at all costs. Fructose is much more difficult for your muscles to utilize for energy which means it is much more likely that it will ultimately get stored as fat before a use for it is found.

Chapter 4: Week 1

Day 1

Breakfast
>Eggs (3 scrambled)
>Grapefruit (1 large)

Snack
>Almonds (25)

Lunch
>Turkey Wrap: This recipe requires 5 minutes to prepare and serves 1

>>*What's in It*
>>- Flour tortilla (1)
>>- Hummus (2 T)
>>- Turkey (2 slices)
>>- Cucumber (.25 sliced)
>>- Tomato (.25 sliced)
>>- Red Onion (.25 sliced)

>>*How's it made*
>>- Combine ingredients as desired serve and enjoy

Snack
>Box of raisins (2 small)

Dinner
>Side Salad with vinegar/olive oil (2 T)
>Pasta and Spicy Chicken: This recipe requires 8 minutes to prepare, 10 minutes to cook and serves 4.

What's in It
- Angel hair pasta (9 oz.)
- Onion (1 cup sliced)
- Dried basil (1 T)
- Parmesan cheese (1 T grated)
- Spinach (10 oz. chopped)
- Chicken breast (6 oz.)
- Black pepper (to taste)
- Salt (to taste)
- Flour (1 tsp.)
- Sour cream (.25 cups)
- Half and half (1 cup)
- Red pepper (.5 tsp. crushed)
- Garlic (1.5 tsp. minced)

How's It Made
- Cook pasta as directed, minus any extra salt or fats. Drain the pasta but make sure to save .25 cups of liquid.
- Coat a skillet and place it on the stove over a burner turned to a high/medium heat.
- Add in the onion and let it cook for 2 minutes before adding in the garlic, red pepper and basil and let everything cook an additional minute.
- In a bowl, combine the flour, sour cream and half and half and mix well.
- Add the results and the reserved liquid to the skillet and let it boil before adding in the remaining ingredients except the pasta and letting everything boil.
- Add in the pasta and let it heat to the desired temperature.

Day 2

Breakfast

    Toast (1 piece)

    Peanut Butter (2 T)

Snack

    Box of raisins (2 small)

Lunch

Chicken Sausage with Peppers: This recipe requires 10 minutes of preparation, 10 minutes to cook and serves 4

What's in It

- Black Pepper (to taste)
- Salt (to taste)
- Basil (.25 cups chopped)
- Marinara sauce (1 cup)
- Worcestershire sauce (1 tsp.)
- Bell peppers (2 sliced)
- Red onion (1 sliced)
- Chicken sausage (1 lb.)
- Olive oil (1 T)

How's it Made

- Add the oil to a skillet before placing the skillet on the stove over a burner set to a high/medium heat.
- Add in the peppers and onions, season as desired and let them cook for 5 minutes.
- Add in the tomato sauce and the Worcestershire Sauce and letting everything cook for an additional 5 minutes. The sausage should be well cooked and the vegetables should be tender
- Top with basil prior to serving.

Snack

    Fat free Greek yogurt (1 serving)

Dinner

    Broccoli (2 cups)

    Miso Salmon: This recipe requires 15 minutes of preparation, 10 minutes to cook and serves 4

        What's in It

- Scallions (2 T)
- Salmon fillet (1.25 lbs. portioned)
- Hot pepper sauce (to taste)
- Ginger (1 T minced)
- Tamari (1 T)
- Mirin (2 T)
- Miso paste (2 T)
- Sesame seeds (1 T)

        How's It Made

- Ensure your broiler is heated and place the oven rack in the top part of the oven.
- Prepare a baking pan by lining it with tinfoil and covering the foil with cooking spray.
- Place the sesame seeds into a skillet and place the skillet on a burner turned to a low heat and let them cook for 3 minutes, stirring all the while.
- In a small bowl, combine the hot pepper sauce, ginger, tamari, soy sauce, mirin and miso and mix well.
- Add the fish to the baking pan with the skin facing the foil. Coat well using the sauce before

broiling the fish for about 7 minutes or until it is opaque in the middle.
- Top with scallions and sesame seeds before serving.

Day 3

Breakfast
  Eggs (2)
  Ham (1 slice)

Snack
  Almonds (25)

Lunch
  White Beans with Pesto and Asparagus: This recipe requires 15 minutes of preparation, 10 minutes to cook and serves 4.
  What's in It-Pesto
  - Black Pepper (to taste)
  - Salt (to taste)
  - Extra virgin olive oil (.25 cups)
  - Lime juice (1 T)
  - Parmesan cheese (.25 cups grated)
  - Garlic (1 clove)
  - Cilantro leaves (1 cup chopped)

  What's in it-meal
  - Coconut oil (1 T)
  - Cherry tomatoes (1 cup sliced)
  - Asparagus (1 lb. chopped)
  - White beans (2 cups)

  How's it Made
  - To form the pesto, simply add the cilantro leaves, garlic, parmesan cheese, lime juice, extra virgin

olive oil, and salt and pepper to a food processor and process well.

- Add the remaining coconut oil to a skillet before placing the skillet on the stove over a burner set to a high/medium heat.
- Add in the asparagus and let it cook until it has softened before mixing in the beans and letting everything cook for 5 minutes.
- Mix in the cherry tomatoes and let everything cook for 2 more minutes before adding in the pesto and cooking for 3 additional minutes.

Snack

String cheese (1)

Dinner

Side Salad with vinegar and olive oil (4 T)

Sweet Potato Fries (1 serving)

Veggie Burger with Whole Wheat Bun: This recipe requires 45 minutes to prepare, 30 minutes to cook and serves 8.

What's in It

- Low sodium soy sauce (1 T)
- Rolled oats (.3 cups quick cooking)
- Pecans (.5 cups toasted, chopped)
- Low fat cheddar cheese (.6 cups shredded)
- Egg (1)
- Oregano (.25 tsp. dried)
- Marjoram (.75 tsp. dried)
- Garlic (1 tsp. minced)
- White button mushrooms (2 cups chopped)
- Onion (1 cup diced)
- Canola oil (1 T)
- Red quinoa (.5 cups)
- Water (1 cup)

How's It Made

- In a saucepan, mix the quinoa and the water before placing the saucepan on the stove and letting it boil. Once it does so, cover it and let it simmer for 15 minutes. Once it is finished cooking, let it sit for 10 minutes, fluff as needed.
- Ensure your oven is heated to 350 degrees Fahrenheit.
- Cover a baking sheet in parchment paper.
- Add oil to a larger saucepan before placing it on top of a burner turned to a medium heat.
- Cook the onion in the saucepan for 5 minutes before adding in the oregano, marjoram, garlic and mushrooms and let everything cook an additional 5 minutes.
- While the second saucepan is cooling, beat the egg in a mixing bowl and then add in the soy sauce, oats, pecans, cheese, mushroom mix and quinoa and mix well.
- Portion out the results into .5 cup servings and place these servings onto the baking sheet before forming them into patties, leaving room for each to expand.
- Place the patties into the microwave and let them bake for 30 minutes

Day 4

Breakfast

Toast (1 slice)
Peanut Butter (2 T)
Fat Free Greek Yogurt (1 serving)

Snack

Snap Peas (15)
Hummus (2 T)

Lunch

Chicken Salad Lettuce Wraps: This recipe requires 10 minutes of preparation, 20 minutes to chill and serves 4

What's in It

- Black Pepper (to taste)
- Salt (to taste)
- Lettuce (4 large leaves)
- Low Fat balsamic vinaigrette (1 cup)
- Fat free Greek Yogurt (2 T plain)
- Cranberries (.25 cups dried)
- Grapes (.5 cups chopped)
- Walnuts (.5 cups toasted)
- Chicken (3 cups cooked, chopped)

How's it Made

- In a mixing bowl, combine the cranberries, grapes, walnuts and chicken and mix well before adding in the Greek yogurt and mixing thoroughly.
- Mix in the vinaigrette and season as desired before refrigerating for at least 20 minutes prior to serving.

Snack

1 Banana

Dinner

Broccoli (2 cups)
Brown rice (1 cup)

Snapper and Pesto: This recipe requires 10 minutes to prepare, 10 minutes to cook and serves 4.

What's in It

- Black pepper (to taste)
- Snapper (24 oz. fillets)
- Salt (.5 tsp.)
- Sugar (1 T)
- Garlic (3 cloves chopped)
- Lime juice (3 T)
- Olive oil (.25 cups)
- Mint leaves (.25 cups packed)
- Parsley (1.5 cups)
- Basil (1.5 cups)

How's It Made

- Add the salt, sugar, garlic, lime juice, oil, mint leaves, parsley and basil to a food processor and process well.
- Add the results to both sides of each fillet and use roughly .5 tsp. per side.
- Season as desired before placing the fish into a grill basket that has been prepared and letting the fish grill for 3.5 minutes on each side.

Day 5

Breakfast

Fat free Greek Yogurt (1 serving)
Grapefruit (1 large)

Snack

Protein Bar (1)

Lunch

    1 apple

    Lean Soufflé: This recipe requires 10 minutes of preparation, 2.5 minutes to cook and serves 4

What's in It

- Black Pepper (to taste)
- Salt (to taste)
- Rice Chex (1 handful crushed)
- Baby spinach (1 handful)
- Eggs (2)
- Extra virgin olive oil (1 T)

How's it Made

- Add the oil to a ramekin and coat well.
- Whisk the eggs together in a small bowl
- Add the crushed Chex to the ramekin and form a layer, follow it up with a layer of spinach and then top with the eggs.
- Stir briefly before adding the ramekin to the microwave and letting it cook for 1 minute before stirring again and letting it cook for another 1 minute and 30 seconds.
- Let cool for 5 minutes prior to eating.

Snack

    Baby carrots (30)
    Hummus (4 T)

Dinner

    Snow peas (2 cups)
    Brown rice (1 cup)
    Spinach with Chicken Parmesan: This recipe requires 20 minutes of preparation, 20 minutes to cook and serves 6.

What's in It

- Whole-grain pasta (6 cups cooked, tossed with oil 2 tsp.)
- Mozzarella cheese (.75 cups shredded)
- Lemon juice (1 tsp.)
- Baby spinach (4 cups)
- Olive oil (2 T+2 tsp.)
- Chicken breast (1.5 lbs. portioned)
- Basil (.25 tsp. dried)
- Black pepper (.25 tsp. ground)
- Salt (.5 tsp. divided)
- Whole wheat flour (2 T)
- Parmesan cheese (3 T grated)
- Honey (.5 tsp.)
- Oregano (.25 tsp.)
- Basil (.25 tsp. dried)
- Whole tomatoes (28 oz.)
- Garlic (2 cloves sliced)
- Extra-virgin olive oil (2 tsp.)

How's It Made

- Ensure your oven is heated to 375 degrees Fahrenheit.
- Coat a baking pan in cooking spray.
- Place a saucepan on the stove over a burner turned to a medium heat before adding in the garlic and oil and letting the garlic cook for half a minute.
- Squeeze each tomato by hand into the pan before mixing in the honey, pepper, salt, oregano and basil. Simmer everything for approximately 20 minutes.

- Mix the basil, pepper, salt, flour and parmesan cheese together before using the results to cover the chicken.
- Add another skillet to the stove over a burner turned to a medium heat before adding in 2 T oil. After the oil begins to simmer, place the chicken in the skillet and cook one side for 6 minutes.
- Add the chicken to the baking pan
- Add the remaining oil to the skillet before adding in the spinach. Let it cook for 2 minutes before swirling in the lemon juice.
- Add the spinach to the top of the chicken and top with sauce and cheese.
- Place the baking pan in the oven and let it cook for 15 minutes.

Day 6
Breakfast
> Eggs (2)
> Vegetable (1)
> Banana (1)

Snack
> String cheese (1)

Lunch
> Sesame Tofu, Scallion and Ginger: This recipe requires 10 minutes of preparation, 5 minutes to cook and serves 2.
> > *What's in It*
> > - Extra-virgin olive oil (2 tsp.)
> > - Salt (to taste)
> > - Black pepper (to taste)

- Smoked paprika (1 tsp.)
- Sesame seeds (2 T)
- Scallions (.25 cups diced)
- Ginger (2 tsp.)
- Tofu (1 cup diced)

How's It Made
- Add the oil to a skillet and place the skillet on the stove over a burner set to a high/medium heat.
- Add in the scallions as well as the ginger and let them cook for 60 seconds before mixing in the tofu and scrambling it.
- Let the tofu cook completely before removing it from the burner and mixing in the smoked paprika, sesame seed and any salt or pepper as desired.

Snack

Cherry Tomatoes (10)
Hummus (2 T)

Dinner

Broccoli (2 cups)
Brown rice (1 cup)
Lemon Chicken with Dill: This recipe requires 30 minutes of active cooking time and serves 4

What's in It
- Lemon juice (1 T)
- Dill (2 T chopped, divided)
- Flour (2 tsp.)
- Low sodium chicken broth (1 cup)
- Garlic (3 cloves minced)
- Onion (.25 cups chopped)
- Extra-virgin olive oil (3 tsp. divided)

- Black pepper (to taste)
- Salt (to taste)
- Chicken breast (1.25 lbs. portioned)

How's It Made
- Add seasoning to the chicken as desired.
- Add 1.5 tsp. of oil to a skillet before placing it on the stove over a burner turned to a high/medium heat. Place the chicken in the skillet and cook each side for 3 minutes. Remove the chicken from the skillet and cover it with foil.
- Turn the burner heat to medium before adding in the rest of the oil as well as garlic and onion before stirring and cooking for 1 minute.
- Combine the lemon juice, dill, flour and broth together before adding the results to the pan and letting everything cook for 3 minutes.
- Add the chicken back to the pan before turning the burner to low and letting everything simmer for 4 minutes.
- Season the sauce as desired and top the chicken with it prior to serving.

Day 7
Breakfast
>Eggs (2)
>Vegetable (1)
>Banana (1)

Snack
>Baby carrots (15)
>Hummus (2 T)

Lunch

Mango Salsa and Pork Tenderloin: Sesame Tofu, Scallion and Ginger: This recipe requires 15 minutes of preparation, 25 minutes to cook and serves 4.

What's in It-Pork

- Extra-virgin olive oil (2 T divided)
- Salt (to taste)
- Black pepper (to taste)
- Pork tenderloin (1.25 lbs.)
- Jerk seasoning (2 T)

What's in It-Salsa

- Lime (1 quartered)
- Salt (to taste)
- Jalapeno (2 tsp. diced)
- Lime juice (1 T)
- Cilantro (.25 cups)
- Red onion (.25 cups)
- Mango (.5 cups)
- Pineapple (1 cup)

How's It Made

- Mix the salt, jerk seasoning and 1 T extra virgin olive oil in a small bowl before coating the pork in the results.
- Place the pork in a sealable plastic bag with the leftover marinade and let it sit in the refrigerator for 30 minutes.
- Combine the pineapple, mango, red onion, cilantro, lime juice, jalapeno and salt together in a food processor and process as desired.
- After the pork has finished marinating, leave it at room temperature to warm for about 15 minutes.
- Add the oil to a skillet and place the skillet on the stove over a burner set to a high/medium heat.

- Once it has warmed completely, add in the pork and let it cook until it is browned on both sides, roughly 2 minutes per side.
- Cover the pan with tinfoil and reduce the heat and continue to let it cook until the internal temperature of the pork reaches 145 degrees Fahrenheit.
- Let the pork cool for 3 minutes prior to serving, top with salsa as desired and garnish with the lime wedge.

Snack

Fat free Greek yogurt (1 serving)

Dinner

Broccoli (2 cups)

Chicken Marengo and Penne: This recipe requires 20 minutes of preparation, 15 minutes to cook and makes 4 servings.

What's in It

- Butter (.5 T)
- Tomatoes (14 oz. chopped)
- Beef broth (.5 cups)
- White wine (.5 cups)
- Tomato paste (2 T)
- Yellow bell pepper (1 seeded, julienned)
- Mushrooms (.5 lbs. sliced)
- Sweet onion (1 sliced)
- Vegetable oil (3 T)
- Flour (.5 cups)
- Black pepper (to taste)
- Salt (to taste)
- Chicken cutlets (3 thinly sliced)

How's It Made

- Season the chicken as desired before coating it in flour.
- Add the oil to a sauté pan before placing the pan over a burner turned to a high/medium heat before adding in the chicken and let it brown for 3 minutes per side.
- Once the chicken has finished browning completely, remove it from the pan before adding in additional oil and mixing in the peppers, mushrooms and onion and letting the cook for 5 minutes, seasoning as needed.
- Mix in the tomato paste, and let it cook for 2 minutes before increasing the heat, mixing in the wine and letting it reduce for 2 minutes.
- Mix in the tomatoes as well as the beef broth and let it start to bubble before mixing in the chicken and letting everything simmer for 3 minutes.
- Before serving, stir in the butter.

Chapter 5: Week 2

Day 1
Breakfast
> Scrambled eggs (3)
> Grapefruit (1 large)

Snack
> Almonds (25)

Lunch
> Chicken Curry Pita: This recipe requires 15 minutes of active cooking time and serves 4.
> > *What's in It*
> > - Sprouts (2 cups)
> > - Pita (4 5-inch, cut in half)
> > - Almonds (.25 cups sliced, toasted)
> > - Cranberries (.5 cups dried)
> > - Celery (1 stalk diced fine)
> > - Pear (1 diced)
> > - Chicken breast (2 cups cubed)
> > - Curry powder (1 T)
> > - Low-fat mayonnaise (.25 cups)
> > - Fat free plain Greek yogurt (6 T)
>
> > *How's It Made*
> > - In a large bowl, mix the curry powder, mayonnaise and yogurt together before adding in the almonds, cranberries, celery, pear and chicken, mix well and season as desired.
> > - Add the results to the pita and top with sprouts.

Snack

> String cheese (1 piece)
> Fat free Greek Yogurt (1 serving)

Dinner

> Snow peas (2 cups)
> Asian Lettuce Wraps: This recipe requires 5 minutes of preparation, 10 minutes to cook and makes 4 servings.

> *What's in It*
>> - Lime (1 wedged)
>> - Cilantro (1 bunch dried)
>> - Mint (1 bunch (dried)
>> - Cucumber (1 peeled, sliced thin)
>> - Lettuce (12 leaves)
>> - Sesame oil (1 tsp.)
>> - Soy sauce (3 T)
>> - Sugar (1 tsp.)
>> - Red pepper flakes (.5 tsp.)
>> - Garlic (2 cloves chopped)
>> - Ginger (2 T chopped)
>> - Scallions (3 sliced)
>> - Red pepper (1 seeded, sliced)
>> - Ground beef (1 lb.)
>> - Vegetable oil (1 T)

> *How's It Made*
>> - Add the oil to a skillet before placing the skillet on the stove over a burner turned to a high/medium heat. Crumble the beef and add it to the skillet to cook for 5 minutes.
>> - Add in the sugar, red pepper flakes, garlic, ginger, scallion and red pepper. Turn the heat off and mix in the sesame oil and soy sauce.
>> - Combine ingredients as desired prior to serving.

Day 2

Breakfast

       Eggs (2)

       Vegetable (1)

       String cheese (1)

Snack

       Fat free Greek Yogurt (1 serving)

       1 banana

Lunch

       Salmon Sammie: This recipe requires 15 minutes of preparation and serves 4.

       What's in It

- Extra-virgin olive oil (1 T)
- Salt (to taste)
- Black pepper (to taste)
- Romaine lettuce (2 large leaves, halved)
- Tomato (8 slices)
- Pumpernickel bread (8 slices toasted)
- Low fat cream cheese (4 T)
- Lemon juice (2 T)
- Red onion (.25 cups minced)
- Salmon (14 oz.)

       How's It Made

- In a mixing bowl, combine the oil, lemon juice, onion and salmon, mix well and season as desired.
- Spread 1 T of the cream cheese on half of the bread slices and then cover this with .5 cups of salmon salad.

- Top with 2 slices of tomato and the remaining bread.

Snack

    Cherry tomatoes (10)
    Hummus (2 T)

Dinner

    Brown Rice (1 cup)
    Broccoli (2 cups)
    Tofu and Broccoli Stir Fry: This recipe requires 30 minutes of active cooking time and makes 4 servings.

What's in It

- Water (3 T)
- Broccoli florets (6 cups)
- Ginger (1 T minced)
- Extra virgin olive oil (2 T divided)
- Salt (.25 tsp.)
- Tofu (14 oz. drained)
- Red pepper flakes (.25 tsp.)
- Sugar (2 T + 1 tsp.)
- Cornstarch (3 T divided)
- Low sodium soy sauce (3 T)
- Dry sherry (.25 cups)
- Vegetable broth (.5 cups)

How's It Made

- In a small bowl, mix the soy sauce, sherry, the broth, red pepper flakes, sugar and 1 T corn starch and combine well.
- Cube tofu and season as desired.
- In a large bowl, place the remainder of the cornstarch before adding in the tofu and coating well.

- Add 1 T oil to a pan and place the pan on the stove over a burner turned to a high/medium heat. Mix in the tofu and let it brown completely.
- Remove the tofu from the skillet before turning the heat to medium and adding in the rest of the oil as well as the ginger and garlic and let it cook for 30 seconds. Add in the water as well as the broccoli before covering the skillet and letting it cook for 3 minutes, stirring regularly.
- Add in the broth mixture and let it thicken for 1 minute.
- Combine all ingredients prior to serving.

Day 3
Breakfast

Eggs (3 scrambled)
Grapefruit (1 large)

Snack

Fat free Greek yogurt (1 serving)
Almonds (25)

Lunch

Charred Tomato, Broccoli and Chicken Salad: This recipe requires 40 minutes of preparation, 20 minutes to cook and serves 6.

What's in It
- Extra-virgin olive oil (2 tsp. + 3T)
- Salt (to taste)
- Black pepper (to taste)
- Lemon juice (.25 cups)
- Chili powder (.5 tsp.)
- Tomatoes (1.5 lbs. halved)
- Broccoli (4 cups florets)

- Chicken breast (1.5 lbs.)

How's It Made
- Add the chicken to a saucepan and fill the saucepan with water so the chicken is covered.
- Add the saucepan to the stove over a burner set to a high heat and let the water simmer. Once it does, cover the pan, reduce the heat and let it cook for 12 minutes.
- Once the chicken has cooled enough to handle, shred it.
- Add a large pot of water to the stove over a burner set to a high heat. After it boils, add in the broccoli and let it cook for 3 minutes.
- Drain the broccoli and refill the pot with cool water.
- Place the skillet on the stove over a burner set to a high heat and coat the halved side of the tomato in oil before placing them in the skillet.
- Let the tomatoes cook for 4 minutes before topping with more oil and charring the other sides as well.
- Remove the tomatoes from the skillet and chop them.
- Add the remaining oil to the skillet without cleaning the skill and mix in the chili powder, pepper and salt and letting them cook for about 30 seconds. Add in the lemon juice and take the pan off of the burner.
- Add the results to a large bowl and mix in the broccoli, chicken and the tomatoes and combine well.

Snack

  String cheese (1)
  Banana (1)

Dinner

  Broccoli (2 cups)
  Sour and Sweet Chicken and Brown Rice: This recipe requires about 30 minutes of active cooking time and makes 4 servings.

  What's in It

  - Water chestnuts (5 oz. drained, sliced)
  - Vegetable medley (6 cups)
  - Low sodium chicken broth (1 cup)
  - Ginger (2 tsp. minced)
  - Garlic (4 cloves minced)
  - Chicken tenders (1 lb. halved)
  - Extra virgin olive oil (2 T)
  - Apricot preserves (2 T)
  - Cornstarch (2 T)
  - Low sodium soy sauce (2 T)
  - Rice vinegar (.25 cups)
  - Instant brown rice (2 cups prepared)

  How's It Made

  - In a small bowl, combine the apricot preserves, cornstarch, soy sauce and vinegar and whisk well.
  - Add 1 T oil to a skillet before placing the skillet on the stove over a burner set to a high/medium heat. Place the chicken in the skillet and let it cook for 2 minutes. After two minutes, stir and then let it cook for an additional 2 minutes. Remove the chicken from the skillet.
  - Add the rest of the oil to the pan before adding in the ginger and garlic and letting them cook for

20 seconds. Mix in the broth and stir while waiting for it to boil. Mix in the vegetables before letting it simmer. Cover the skillet and let everything cook for 4 minutes.

- Add in the chicken and the water chestnuts before adding in the sauce. Let it thicken for 1 minute and mix with rice prior to serving.

Day 4

Breakfast

Toast (1 slice)
Peanut Butter (2 T)

Snack

Raisins (2 small boxes)

Lunch

Sun Dried Tomato, Corn and Turkey Wrap: This recipe requires 20 minutes of preparation and serves 4.

What's in It

- Extra-virgin olive oil (2 T)
- Salt (to taste)
- Black pepper (to taste)
- Romaine Lettuce (2 cups)
- Whole wheat tortillas (4)
- Turkey (8 oz. sliced)
- Red wine vinegar (1 T)
- Sun-dried tomatoes (.25 cups chopped)
- Tomato (.5 cups chopped)
- Corn (1 cup kernels)

- In a mixing bowl, combine the red wine vinegar, the extra virgin olive oil, the sun dried tomatoes, the regular tomatoes and the corn and mix well.
- Add the turkey and lettuce to the tortillas before filling them with the mixture from the bowl.

Snack

Protein bar (1)

Dinner

Broccoli (2 cups)

Brown Rice (1 cup)

Chicken with Lime and Cilantro: This recipe requires 10 minutes of preparation, 40 minutes to cook and makes 8 servings.

What's in It

- Cilantro (.25 cups chopped)
- Lime juice (2 limes)
- Low sodium chicken broth (1 cup)
- Garlic (2 cloves minced)
- Unsalted butter (4 T divided)
- Black pepper (to taste)
- Salt (to taste)
- Paprika (1 tsp.)
- Basil (1 tsp. dried)
- Oregano (2 tsp. dried)
- Chicken thighs (8)
- Brown sugar (8 tsp. divided)

How's It Made

- Ensure you oven is heated to 400 degrees Fahrenheit.

- Coat the chicken with a mixture of sugar, pepper, salt, paprika, basil and oregano.
- Add 2 T butter to a skillet before placing the skillet on the stove over a burner turned to a high/medium heat. Place the chicken in the skillet with the skin touching the skillet and sear each side for approximately 2 minutes until browned.
- Drain the fat from the skillet and remove the chicken from the skillet.
- Add the rest of the butter to the skillet before adding in the garlic and letting it cook for 1 minute, stirring regularly. Add in the broth, cilantro and lime juice before letting it boil and then turning the heat down and letting it simmer for 5 minutes.
- Add the chicken back into the skillet before placing the skillet in the oven and letting it cook for about 25 minutes or until the center of the chicken reaches 165 degrees Fahrenheit.

Day 5
Breakfast
>Eggs (2)
>Vegetable (1)
>Grapefruit (1 large)

Snack
>Fat Free Greek Yogurt (1 serving)
>Banana (1)

Lunch

Crab Roll: This recipe requires 20 minutes of preparation and serves 4.

What's in It

- Salt (to taste)
- Black pepper (to taste)
- Whole wheat pita (4)
- Red lettuce (4 leaves)
- Crabmeat (2 cups cooked)
- Chives (.25 cups sliced, divided)
- Celery (.25 cups chopped)
- Shallot (.25 cups chopped)
- Hot sauce (10 dashes)
- Lemon juice (3 T)
- Lemon zest (1 T grated)
- Fat free mayonnaise (.25 cups)

How's It Made

- In a mixing bowl, combine the salt, pepper, hot sauce, lemon juice, lemon zest and mayonnaise together and whisk well.
- Add in 3 T chives, celery and shallot and mix well before adding in the crab and mixing gently.
- Add the lettuce to the pita and fill each with the crab mixture, top with the remaining chives.

Snack

Baby carrots (15)
Hummus (2 T)

Dinner

Brown rice (1 cup)
Broccoli (2 cups)

Dill Sauce and Salmon: This recipe requires 15 minutes of preparation time and makes 4 servings.

What's in It

- Capers (1 T chopped)
- Dill (2 T chopped)
- Lemon juice (2 T)
- Sour cream (.5 cups)
- Green beans (1 lb. trimmed)
- Black pepper (to taste)
- Salt (to taste)
- Salmon fillet (24 oz. portioned)
- Extra Virgin Olive Oil (1 T)

How's It Made

- Add the oil to your skillet before placing the skillet on the stove over a medium heat.
- Season the salmon as desired before adding it to the skillet and letting it cook for 5 minutes on each side and ensuring the center is opaque.
- While the fish is cooking, place a steamer basket into a saucepan and let 1 inch of water in the pan begin to boil. Add the beans and cover the pot to let them cook for 4 minutes.
- Mix together the capers, dill, lemon juice, sour cream and pepper and salt as desired and top the salmon prior to serving.

Day 6

Breakfast

Ham (1 slice)
Eggs (2)
Grapefruit (1 medium)

Snack

    Almonds (25)

    String cheese (1)

Lunch

White Bean Salad with Chicken: This recipe requires 25 minutes of preparation and serves 4.

What's in It-Salad

- Salt (to taste)
- Black pepper (to taste)
- Radicchio leaves (2 cups torn)
- Romaine lettuce (2 cups torn)
- Basil (1 cup chopped coarse)
- Sun dried tomatoes (.3 cups chopped)
- Feta cheese (.25 cups diced)
- Celery (1.5 cups diced)
- Zucchini (2 cups diced)
- Chicken breast (2.5 cups diced)
- White beans (15 oz.)

What's in It-Vinaigrette

- Dijon mustard (1 T)
- White wine vinegar (.25 cups)
- Orange juice (6 T)
- Extra virgin olive oil (5 T)
- Salt (.25 tsp.)
- Garlic (1 clove peeled, smashed)

How's It Made

- To create the vinaigrette, start by mashing the garlic along with .25 tsp. salt in a small bowl to create a paste.
- Add in 5 T oil and mix well before mixing in the orange juice, mustard, vinegar and combine

thoroughly. Add up to 4 more Tablespoons of juice to cut the flavor as needed.

- In a large bowl, combine the sun dried tomatoes, cheese, celery, zucchini, chicken and white beans and mix well. Add in .75 cups vinaigrette and the basil, season as needed and mix well.
- Add all of the ingredients to a salad bowl and mix well prior to serving.

Snack

Cherry Tomatoes (10)

Hummus (2 T)

Dinner

Broccoli (2 cups)

Poblanos Stuffed with Barley: This recipe requires 10 minutes of preparation, 55 minutes to cook and makes 6 servings.

What's in It

- Queso fresco (.5 cups crumbled)
- Low fat Monterey Jack cheese (3 slices halved)
- Low fat white cheddar (2 oz. grated)
- Poblano peppers (6 large)
- Slat (.25 tsp.)
- Whole peeled tomatoes (28 oz. crushed)
- Garlic (3 cloves minced)
- Chili powder (1 tsp. divided)
- Kale (1 bunch chopped)
- Barley (1.5 cups soaked, drained)
- Onion (1 diced)
- Extra virgin olive oil (3 T)

How's It Made

- Add 1 T oil to a saucepan and place it over a burner turned to a medium heat. Place the onion in the pan and let it cook for 5 minutes before adding in 3.75 cups water and the barley and letting it cook for 30 minutes before adding in the cheddar cheese, kale and half of the chili powder.

- While the barely is cooking, place the rest of the oil into a heavy pot before placing the pot on the stove over a burner turned to a medium heat. Add in the garlic and let it cook for 3 minutes before adding in the tomatoes, the rest of the chili powder and the salt before letting the pot boil. Let the pot simmer for 30 minutes, covered on a low heat.
- Ensure your broiler is heated and positioned in the middle of the oven.
- Cut the tops off of the peppers and remove the innards but save the tops. Add the barley mix to the peppers and place the tops back on before placing them in a baking dish and broiling them for 20 minutes, turning at the 10-minute mark.
- At this point, put the tomato sauce in the pan as well. Add .5 slices of the Monterey Jack cheese to the top of each pepper. Melt the cheese by broiling for 1 minute.
- Top with queso fresco prior to serving.

Day 7

Breakfast
    Toast (1 slice)
    Peanut butter (2 T)
    Grapefruit (1 large)

Snack

    Raisins (2 small boxes)

    String cheese (1)

Lunch

Tarragon chicken salad: This recipe requires 15 minutes of preparation, 30 minutes to cook and serves 8.

What's in It

- Salt (to taste)
- Black pepper (to taste)
- Red grapes (1.5 cups halved)
- Celery (1.5 cups sliced)
- Tarragon (1 T)
- Fat free mayonnaise (.5 cups)
- Low fat sour cream (.6 cups)
- Walnuts (.3 cups chopped)
- Low sodium chicken broth (1 cup)
- Chicken breast (2 lbs.)

How's It Made

- Ensure your oven is heated to 450 degrees Fahrenheit.
- Place the chicken into a glass baking dish so that it is spread in a single layer and then add in the broth.
- Let the chicken bake for 30 minutes or until its internal temperature reads 170 degrees Fahrenheit.
- Cube the chicken once it has cooled.
- Place the walnuts onto a baking sheet and toast them in the oven for approximately 6 minutes before letting them cool.
- In a mixing bowl, combine the pepper, salt, tarragon, mayonnaise and sour cream together

before adding in the walnuts, chicken, grapes and celery and coating well.

- Chill for 1 hour prior to serving.

Snack

Baby carrots (15)
Hummus (2 T)

Dinner

Side salad with vinegar and olive oil (2 T)
Baja Fish Tacos: This recipe requires 5 minutes of preparation, 8 minutes to cook and makes 4 servings.

What's in It

- Limes (2 wedged)
- Salsa (to taste)
- Avocado (.5 diced, pitted)
- Corn tortillas (8)
- Cilantro (3 T)
- Salt (.5 tsp.)
- Lime juice (1 T)
- Green cabbage (2 cups sliced)
- Fajita seasoning (2 tsp.)
- Mahi Mahi (.75 lbs.)

How's It Made

- Prepare the grill and heat it to a medium heat.
- Season the fish as desired before adding it to the grill and letting each side cook for 3 minutes.
- Combine the cilantro, salt, lime juice and cabbage together in a bowl.
- Combine all ingredients prior to serving.

Chapter 6: Week 3

Day 1
Breakfast
       Eggs (2)
       Vegetable (1)
       Grapefruit (1 large)

Snack
       Cherry Tomatoes (10)
       Hummus (2 T)

Lunch
       Tofu Peanut Wrap: This recipe requires 10 minutes of preparation and serves 1.

       What's in It
- Snow peas (8 sliced)
- Red bell pepper (.25 cups sliced)
- Tofu (2 oz. baked, sliced)
- Wheat tortilla (1)
- Peanut Sauce (1 T)

       How's It Made
- . Add all of the ingredients to the tortilla, wrap and serve.

Snack
       Fat free Greek yogurt (1 serving)

Dinner
       Broccoli (2 cups)

Fettuccine with Peas and Shrimp: This recipe requires 10 minutes of preparation, 1 minutes to cook and makes 3 servings.

What's in It

- Parmesan cheese (to taste)
- Peas (3 T)
- Rosemary (.5 tsp. crushed)
- Garlic (1 tsp. minced)
- Tomatoes (.25 cups chopped)
- Shrimp (.3 cups)
- Extra Virgin olive oil (1 T)
- Whole wheat pasta (1 package prepared)

How's It Made

- Add the oil to a skillet before adding in the rosemary, garlic and tomatoes and letting them cook for 5 minutes, stirring twice per minute.
- Add in the peas and then cook and stir for 2 minutes.
- Combine all of the ingredients and top with the cheese prior to serving.

Day 2

Breakfast

Eggs (3 scrambled)
Grapefruit (1 large)

Snack

String cheese (1)

Lunch

Turkey Lettuce Wrap: This recipe requires 30 minutes of preparation and serves 6.

What's in It
- Sesame oil (2 tsp.)
- Salt (to taste)
- Black pepper (to taste)
- Carrot (1 shredded)
- Cilantro (.5 cups chopped)
- Basil (.5 cups chopped)
- Mint (.5 cups chopped)
- Boston lettuce (2 heads separated leaves)
- Five spice powder (1 tsp.)
- Hoisin sauce (2 T)
- Low sodium chicken broth (.5 cups reduced)
- Water chestnuts (8 oz. chopped)
- Red bell pepper (1 diced fine)
- Ginger (1 T minced)
- Ground turkey (1 lb.)
- Instant brown rice (.5 cups)
- Water (.5 cup)

How's It Made
- Fill a small saucepan with water and place it on the stove over a burner set to a high heat and let the water boil. Add in the rice and let it cook for 5 minutes and remove the saucepan from the burner.
- Add the oil to a skillet and place it on the stove over a burner set to a medium heat. Add in the ginger and crumble in the turkey before letting it cook for 6 minutes.
- Add in the rice, salt, pepper, five spice powder, hoisin sauce, broth, water chestnuts, mint, basil, cilantro, bell pepper and let everything cook for 1 minute.

- Add the turkey mix, carrots and herbs to each piece of lettuce and roll it like a burrito.

Snack

Almonds (25)

Dinner

Brown rice (1 cup)

Veggie Stir Fry: This recipe requires 15 minutes of preparation, 5 minutes to cook and makes 6 servings.

What's in It

- Sesame oil (2 T)
- Snow peas (.5 cups)
- Salt (.25 tsp.)
- Black pepper (.25 tsp.)
- Mung bean sprouts (1 cup)
- Bok choy (2 cups sliced)
- Teriyaki sauce (.5 cups)
- Garlic (1 clove minced)
- Eggplant (1 chopped)
- Broccoli (1 cup florets)
- Yellow squash (1 cup sliced)
- Red onion (.5 cups sliced thin)
- Yellow bell pepper (seeded, cored, julienned)
- Extra virgin olive oil (2 T)

How's It Made

- Add the oil to a skillet before adding the skillet to the stove over a burner turned to a high heat. Once the skillet is almost smoking, mix in the onion and peppers before adding in the garlic eggplant, broccoli, squash and the sauce.

- Stir for 2 minutes before adding in the seasoning, sprouts and bok choy and stirring for an additional 2 minutes.
- Remove the skillet from the heat and add in the sesame oil and snow peas prior to serving.

Day 3
Breakfast

Oatmeal (1 serving)

Grapefruit (1 large)

Snack

String cheese (1)

Lunch

Cobb Salad: This recipe requires 15 minutes of preparation, 25 minutes to cook and serves 4.

What's in It

- Extra-virgin olive oil (3 T)
- Salt (to taste)
- Black pepper (to taste)
- Blue cheese (.5 cups crumbles)
- Avocado (1 diced)
- Cucumber (1 sliced, seeded)
- Tomatoes (2 diced)
- Eggs (2)
- Cooked chicken breast (8 oz.)
- Salad greens (10 cups)
- Dijon mustard (1 T)
- Shallot (2 T minced)
- White wine vinegar (3 T)

How's It Made

- Start by poaching the chicken breast. Add it to a skillet before covering it in salted water. Add the skillet to the stove over a burner set to a high/medium heat and let it boil.
- Once it does, turn the burner to low and let it simmer for 10 minutes or until the chicken reaches 165 degrees Fahrenheit internally.
- Let the chicken cool and then shred it.
- Place the eggs in a saucepan and cover them with 1 inch of water. Add the pan to the stove over a burner set to a high/medium heat. Once the pan simmers, reduce the heat and let it slightly simmer 10 minutes.
- Drain the eggs and cover them with cool water. Once they have cooled, peel and chop them.
- In a small bowl, combine the salt, pepper, mustard, shallot and vinegar and mix well.
- In a large bowl, combine the salad greens with 50 percent of the dressing and coat well.
- Plate everything and top with the remaining dressing prior to serving.

Snack

Fat free Greek Yogurt (1 serving)

Dinner

Side salad with vinegar and olive oil (2 T)
Broccoli (2 cups)
Balsamic chicken: This recipe requires 10 minutes of preparation, 25 minutes to cook and makes 6 servings.

What's in It

- Thyme (.5 tsp. dried)
- Rosemary (1 tsp. dried)
- Oregano (1 tsp. dried)

- Basil (1 tsp. dried)
- Balsamic vinegar (.5 cups)
- Tomatoes (14.5 oz. diced)
- Onion (1 sliced thin)
- Extra virgin olive oil (2 T)
- Black pepper (to taste)
- Garlic salt (1 tsp.)
- Chicken breast (3 halved)

How's It Made
- Season the chicken as desired.
- Add the oil to the skillet before placing the skillet on the stove over a burner set to a medium heat. Add in the chicken and let it cook for 3 minutes per side.
- Add in the onion and let everything cook an additional 3 minutes.
- Add in the vinegar and tomatoes on top of the chicken before adding in the thyme, rosemary, oregano and basil. Let everything simmer for 15 minutes, the chicken should reach a temperature of 165 degrees Fahrenheit.

Day 4

Breakfast
> Ham (1 slice)
> Eggs (2)
> Grapefruit (1 medium)

Snack
> Fat Free Greek Yogurt
> 1 banana

Lunch

Tuna Panini: This recipe requires 25 minutes of preparation and serves 4.

What's in It

- Extra-virgin olive oil (2 tsp.)
- Salt (to taste)
- Black pepper (to taste)
- Wholegrain bread (8 slices)
- Lemon juice (1 tsp.)
- Capers (1 tsp. chopped)
- Kalamata olives (1 T chopped, pitted)
- Red onion (2 T minced)
- Artichoke hearts (2 T chopped)
- Feta cheese (.25 cups crumbled)
- Plum tomato (1 chopped)
- Light tuna (12 oz. chunked)

How's It Made

- Flake the tuna in a bowl with the help of a fork. Mix in the pepper, salt, lemon juice, capers, olives, onion, artichokes, feta and tomato and combine well.
- Place .5 cups of the tuna mixture on half of the slices. And top the sandwiches.
- Add the oil to a skillet and place the skillet on the stove over a burner set to a high/medium heat. Add 2 panni to the skillet at a time, and cook the first side for 2 minutes, reduce the heat to low/medium and cook the other side for 2 minutes.
- Add additional oil for the second set of sandwiches as needed.

Snack

String cheese (1)

Dinner

Broccoli (2 cups)
Brown rice (1 cup)
Swai Fillet: This recipe requires 10 minutes of preparation, 15 minutes to cook and makes 4 servings.

What's in It

- Paprika (1 tsp.)
- Black pepper (1 tsp.)
- Salt (1 tsp.)
- Garlic (1 tsp. minced)
- Cilantro (1 T)
- Lemon juice (1 T)
- Dry white wine (.25 cups)
- Margarine (2 T)
- Swai fish fillet (16 oz. portioned)

How's It Made

- Ensure your oven is heated to 350 degrees Fahrenheit.
- Coat a baking sheet in cooking spray and add in the fillets.
- Add the margarine to a saucepan before adding the pan to the stove over a burner turned to a medium heat. Add in the pepper, salt, garlic, cilantro, lemon juice and white wine and let it simmer for 2 minutes.
- Add in the paprika and ensure the fish is well covered in the sauce before adding the pan to the oven and letting it cook for 10 minutes.

Day 5

Breakfast

      Toast (1 slice)

      Peanut butter (2 T)

      Grapefruit (1 medium)

Snack

      Banana (1)

      Box of raisins (1 small)

Lunch

      Red Lentil Curry Soup: This recipe requires 15 minutes of preparation, 45 minutes to cook and serves 6.

      What's in It

- Extra-virgin olive oil (1 T)
- Salt (to taste)
- Black pepper (to taste)
- Fat free plain Greek yogurt (.3 cups)
- Mango chutney (2 T)
- Lemon juice (2 T)
- Cilantro (3 T)
- Low sodium chicken broth (8 cups)
- Red lentils (1.5 cups)
- Bay leaves (2)
- Cumin (1 tsp. ground)
- Cinnamon (1 tsp.)
- Curry powder (1.5 T)
- Jalapeno (1 seeded, minced)
- Ginger (2 T minced)
- Garlic (3 cloves minced)
- Onion (1 chopped)

How's It Made

- Add the oil to a stockpot and place the pot on the stove over a burner set to a medium heat. Add in the onion and let it cook for 3 minutes before adding in the bay leaves, cumin, cinnamon, curry powder, jalapeno, ginger and garlic. Stir and let it cook for 5 minutes.
- Add in the chicken broth as well as the lentils and let the pot boil before turning the heat to low, covering the pot part way and letting it simmer for 45 minutes.
- Remove the bay leaves and add in the cilantro, chutney and lemon juice before seasoning as desired.
- Add the yogurt to each bowl prior to serving.

Snack

Baby carrots (15)
Hummus (2 T)

Dinner

Side salad with vinegar and olive oil (2 T)
Bean Quesadilla: This recipe requires 15 minutes of active preparation time and makes 4 servings.

What's in It

- Avocado (1 diced)
- Extra virgin olive oil (2 tsp.)
- Whole wheat tortillas (4)
- Salsa (.5 cups)
- Monterey Jack cheese (.5 cups shredded)
- Black beans (15 oz.)

How's It Made

- In a mixing bowl, combine .25 cups salsa with the Monterey Jack cheese and the black beans before mixing well.
- Add the results to the tortillas before folding them in half.
- Add 1 tsp. of extra virgin olive oil to a skillet and place the skillet on the stove over an oven turned to a medium heat. Cook each side of each quesadilla for 2 minutes. 1 tsp. of olive oil will cook 2 quesadillas.

Day 6
Breakfast

    Eggs (3 scrambled)
    Grapefruit (1 large)

Snack

    Almonds (25)

Lunch

    Spicy Chicken Pitas: This recipe requires 15 minutes of preparation,15 minutes to cook and serves 4.

    What's in It
- Extra-virgin olive oil (2 T)
- Salt (to taste)
- Black pepper (to taste)
- Red onion (.25 cups sliced thin)
- Tomato (1 sliced)
- Romaine lettuce (1 cup shredded)
- Whole wheat pitas (4 warmed)
- Lemon juice (2 tsp.)
- Cilantro (1 T chopped)
- Mint (1 T chopped)
- Fat free plain Greek Yogurt (.75 cups)

- Cucumber (1 cup sliced thin)
- Garam masala (1.5 tsp.)
- Chicken breast (1 lb. trimmed)

How's It Made
- Heat your grill to a high/medium temperature and oil the rack as needed.
- Coat the chicken with the garam masala, salt and pepper as needed. Grill each side of the chicken for approximately 5 minutes until the internal temperature reads 165 degree Fahrenheit.
- Remove the chicken from the grill and let it cool for 5 minutes before slicing.
- In a small bowl, combine the pepper, salt, remaining garam masala, lemon juice, cilantro, mint, Greek yogurt and cucumber and mix well.
- Split the pitas and fill them with the onion, tomato, lettuce, yogurt sauce and chicken.

Snack

String cheese (1 piece)

Dinner

Broccoli (2 cups)
Brown rice (1 cup)
Chicken Dijon: This recipe requires 5 minutes of preparation, 10 minutes to cook and makes 2 servings.

What's in It
- Olive oil (1 T)
- Black pepper (.5 tsp.)
- Salt (.5 tsp.)
- Parsley (6 sprigs)
- Dijon mustard (2 tsp.)
- Garlic (1 clove crushed)

- Chicken breast (8 oz. portioned)

How's It Made
- Heat your grill to a medium heat.
- In a small bowl, mix together the pepper, salt, parsley mustard and garlic and combine well.
- Coat the chicken in the mixture.
- Grill the chicken for 5 minutes per side, the chicken's internal temperature should be 165 degrees Fahrenheit.

Day 7
Breakfast
Eggs (2)
Vegetable (1)
Grapefruit (1 medium)

Snack
Protein bar (1)

Lunch

Turkey Tostada: This recipe requires 30 minutes of preparation, 10 minutes to cook and serves 4.
What's in It
- Extra-virgin olive oil (2 tsp.)
- Salt (to taste)
- Black pepper (to taste)
- Monterey Jack cheese (.5 cups)
- Romaine lettuce (1 cup shredded)
- Low fat sour cream (2 T)
- Salsa (.25 cups)
- Avocado (1 pitted)
- Corn tortillas (8)
- Turkey (3 cups shredded, cooked)

- Onion (1 sliced thin)
- Tomatoes (14 oz. diced)
- Jalapeno (1 chopped, seeded)

How's It Made
- Ensure your oven is heated to 375 degrees Fahrenheit. Set your oven racks to the lower and upper thirds.
- Boil the tomatoes using their own canned juice in a saucepan placed on a burner turned to a medium heat. Mix in the onion and let it cook for 15 minutes before mixing in the turkey and letting it cook for 1.5 minutes.
- Add the oil to both sides of the tortillas and place them on a pair of baking sheets.
- Place the baking sheets in the oven and bake for 5 minutes, turn the sheets and bake for another 5 minutes.
- In a small bowl, smash the avocado and mix in the cilantro, sour cream and salsa and mix well.
- Top the tortillas with avocado, the turkey mix, cheese and lettuce prior to serving.

Snack

Raisins (2 boxes)

Dinner

Brown rice (1 cup)

Edamame and Salmon: This recipe requires 20 minutes of preparation, 8 minutes to cook and makes 4 servings.

What's in It
- Edamame (1.3 cups cooked)
- Black sesame seed (.25 tsp.)
- Honey (2 tsp.)

- Low fat soy sauce (2 tsp.)
- Lime juice (2 tsp.)
- Salmon fillet (24 oz. portioned)
- Black pepper (to taste)
- Salt (to taste)
- Ginger (1 tsp.)
- Extra virgin olive oil (2 tsp.)
- Scallions (2)
- Cilantro leaves (.25 cups packed)

How's It Made

- Ensure your grill is heated to a high/medium heat and is oiled.
- In a bowl, combine the ginger, oil, scallion and cilantro before seasoning as desired.
- Cut a 3-inch slit in the bottom of each fillet and add the mixture to each before seasoning the fish as needed.
- In a small bowl, combine the honey, soy and lime juice.
- Place the fish on the grill and let each side cook for 4 minutes. Top the fish with the lime, soy and honey sauce.

Chapter 7: Week 4

Day 1

Breakfast
>   Eggs (3 scrambled)
>   Grapefruit (1 large)

Snack
>   String Cheese (1)

Lunch
>   Chicken Curry Pita (Week 2, Day 1)

Snack
>   Fat free Greek yogurt (1 serving)

Dinner
>   Side Salad with vinegar/olive oil (2 T)
>   Pasta and Spicy Chicken (Week 1, Day 1)

Day 2

Breakfast
>   Toast (1 piece)
>   Peanut Butter (2 T)

Snack
>   Box of raisins (2 small)

Lunch
>   Salmon Sammie (Week 2, Day 2)

Snack

Almonds (25)

Dinner
Snow peas (2 cups)
Asian Lettuce Wraps (Week 2, Day 1)

Day 3

Breakfast
Eggs (2)
Ham (1 slice)

Snack
Snap Peas (15)
Hummus (2 T)

Lunch
Charred Tomato, Broccoli and Chicken Salad (Week 2, Day 3)

Snack
1 Banana

Dinner
Brown Rice (1 cup)
Broccoli (2 cups)
Tofu and Broccoli Stir Fry (Week 2, Day 2)

Day 4

Breakfast
Eggs (2)
Vegetable (1)
Banana (1)

Snack

Baby carrots (30)

Hummus (4 T)

Lunch

Sun Dried Tomato, Corn and Turkey Wrap (Week 2, Day 4)

Snack

Fat free Greek yogurt (1 serving)

Dinner

Broccoli (2 cups)

Brown rice (1 cup)

Chicken Dijon (Week 3, Day 6)

Day 5

Breakfast

Fat free Greek Yogurt (1 serving)

Grapefruit (1 large)

Snack

1 Banana

Lunch

Crab Roll (Week 2, Day 5)

Snack

Snap Peas (15)

Hummus (2 T)

Dinner

Broccoli (2 cups)

Brown Rice (1 cup)

Chicken with Lime and Cilantro (Week 2, Day 4)

Day 6

Breakfast
>Scrambled eggs (3)
>Grapefruit (1 large)

Snack
>Protein bar (1)

Lunch
>White Bean Salad with Chicken (Week 2, Day 6)

Snack
>Almonds (25)

Dinner
>Side Salad with vinegar and olive oil (4 T)
>Sweet Potato Fries (1 serving)
>Veggie Burger with Whole Wheat Bun (Week 1, Day 3)

Day 7

Breakfast
>Eggs (2)
>Vegetable (1)
>String cheese (1)

Snack
>Box of raisins (2 small)

Lunch
>Tarragon chicken salad (Week 2, Day 7)

Snack
>Fat free Greek yogurt (1 serving)

Dinner

    Broccoli (2 cups)

    Sour and Sweet Chicken and Brown Rice (Week 2, Day 3)

Chapter 8: Week 5

Day 1

Breakfast
> Eggs (3 scrambled)
> Grapefruit (1 large)

Snack
> Fat free Greek yogurt (1 serving)

Lunch
> Turkey Wrap (Week 1, Day 1)

Snack
> Snap Peas (15)
> Hummus (2 T)

Dinner
> Broccoli (2 cups)
> Fettuccine with Peas and Shrimp (Week 3, Day 1)

Day 2

Breakfast
> Toast (1 slice)
> Peanut Butter (2 T)

Snack
> Almonds (25)

Lunch
> Chicken Sausage with Peppers (Week 1, Day 2)

Snack

    Baby carrots (30)

    Hummus (4 T)

Dinner

    Broccoli (2 cups)

    Miso Salmon (Day 2, Week 1)

Day 3

Breakfast

    Eggs (2)

    Vegetable (1)

    Grapefruit (1 large)

Snack

    1 Banana

Lunch

    White Beans with Pesto and Asparagus (Week 1, Day 3)

Snack

    Box of raisins (2 small)

Dinner

    Brown rice (1 cup)

    Broccoli (2 cups)

    Dill Sauce and Salmon (Week 2, Day 5)

Day 4

Breakfast

    Ham (1 slice)

    Eggs (2)

    Grapefruit (1 medium)

Snack

    Fat free Greek yogurt (1 serving)

Lunch

    Chicken Salad Lettuce Wraps (Week 1, Day 4)

Snack

    Baby carrots (30)

    Hummus (4 T)

Dinner

    Brown rice (1 cup)

    Veggie Stir Fry (Week 3, Day 2)

Day 5

Breakfast

    Toast (1 slice)

    Peanut butter (2 T)

    Grapefruit (1 large)

Snack

    Almonds (25)

Lunch

    Lean Soufflé (Week 1, Day 5)

Snack

    Snap Peas (15)

    Hummus (2 T)

Dinner

    Broccoli (2 cups)

    Brown rice (1 cup)

Snapper and Pesto (Week 1, Day 4)

Day 6

Breakfast
    Eggs (2)
    Vegetable (1)
    Grapefruit (1 large)

Snack
    Fat free Greek yogurt (1 serving)

Lunch
    Sesame Tofu, Scallion and Ginger (Week 1, Day 6)

Snack
    1 Banana

Dinner
    Broccoli (2 cups)
    Brown Rice (1 cup)
    Poblanos Stuffed with Barley (Week 2, Day 6)

Day 7

Breakfast
    Eggs (3 scrambled)
    Grapefruit (1 large)

Snack
    Box of raisins (2 small)

Lunch
    Mango Salsa and Pork Tenderloin (Week 1, Day 7)

Snack

       Baby carrots (30)

       Hummus (4 T)

Dinner

       Side salad with vinegar and olive oil (2 T)

       Broccoli (2 cups)

       Balsamic chicken (Week 3, Day 3)

Chapter 9: Week 6

Day 1

Breakfast
> Oatmeal (1 serving)
> Grapefruit (1 large)

Snack
> Banana (1)
> Fat free Greek yogurt (1 serving)

Lunch
> Tofu Peanut Wrap (Week 4, Day 1)

Snack
> Box of raisins (2 small)

Dinner
> Snow peas (2 cups)
> Brown rice (1 cup)
> Spinach with Chicken Parmesan (Week 1, Day 5)

Day 2

Breakfast
> Ham (1 slice)
> Eggs (2)
> Grapefruit (1 medium)

Snack
> Snap Peas (15)
> Hummus (2 T)

Lunch

     Turkey Lettuce Wrap (Week 3, Day 2)

Snack

     Fat free Greek yogurt (1 serving)

Dinner

     Side salad with vinegar and olive oil (2 T)
     Baja Fish Tacos (Week 2, Day 7)

Day 3

Breakfast

     Toast (1 slice)
     Peanut butter (2 T)
     Grapefruit (1 medium)

Snack

     Almonds (25)

Lunch

     Cobb Salad (Week 3, Day 3)

Snack

     Baby carrots (30)
     Hummus (4 T)

Dinner

     Broccoli (2 cups)
     Brown rice (1 cup)
     Swai Fillet (Week 3, Day 4)

Day 4

Breakfast

Eggs (3 scrambled)
Grapefruit (1 large)

Snack

1 Banana

Lunch

Tuna Panini (Week 3, Day 4)

Snack

Cherry Tomatoes (10)
Hummus (2 T)

Dinner

Broccoli (2 cups)
Brown rice (1 cup)
Lemon Chicken with Dill (Week 1, Day 6)

Day 5

Breakfast

Eggs (2)
Vegetable (1)
Grapefruit (1 medium)

Snack

Box of raisins (2 small)

Lunch

Red Lentil Curry Soup (Week 3, Day 5)

Snack

Baby carrots (30)
Hummus (4 T)

Dinner
>Side salad with vinegar and olive oil (2 T)
>Bean Quesadilla (Week 3, Day 5)

Day 6

Breakfast
>Eggs (3 scrambled)
>Grapefruit (1 large)

Snack
>Almonds (25)
>Banana (1)

Lunch
>Spicy Chicken Pitas (Week 3, Day 6)

Snack
>Snap Peas (15)
>Hummus (2 T)

Dinner
>Broccoli (2 cups)
>Chicken Marengo and Penne (Week 1, Day 7)

Day 7

Breakfast
>Toast (1 piece)
>Peanut Butter (2 T)

Snack
>Almonds (25)

Lunch

Turkey Tostada (Week 3, Day 7)

Snack

Fat free Greek yogurt (1 serving)
Almonds (25)

Dinner

Brown rice (1 cup)
Edamame and Salmon (Week 3, Day 7)

Conclusion

Thank you again for downloading this book! I hope this book was able to help you to learn everything you need to in order to take advantage of all of the opportunities that sticking with a lean lifestyle offers. It is important to keep up the good work now that you are at the end of your 6-week struggle. Remember how hard you had to fight to get here and don't let it all go to waste. Being lean is a journey, not a destination, and your journey is just beginning.

The next step is to stop reading already and use the recipes you have learned as a blueprint for future culinary adventures. Remember to stick with clean ingredients as strictly as possible and you can't go wrong. Happy eating!

Finally, if you enjoyed this book, then I'd like to ask you for a favor, would you be kind enough to leave a review for this book on Amazon? It'd be greatly appreciated!

Special Invitation!

If you liked what you read and would like to read high quality books, get free bonuses, and get notified first of **FREE EBOOKS,** then join the official Xcension Publishing Company Book Club! Membership is free, but space is limited!

You can join the Book Club by visiting the link below:

http://www.xcensionpublishing.com/book-club